Different Minds
Living with ALZHEIMER DISEASE

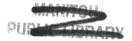

Presented By:

Alzheimer *Society*
MANITOBA

January 2006
HELPLINE: 1-800-378-6699
Telephone: 1-204-943-6622
Web site: www.alzheimer.mb.ca

Different Minds

**Living with
ALZHEIMER DISEASE**

LORNA DREW and LEO C. FERRARI

All royalties from the sale of *Different Minds* will be used to support the Alzheimer Society of Canada research program.

Edited by Sabine Campbell.
Cover photo: Stockbyte Photography.
Cover and interior design by Julie Scriver.
Printed in Canada.
10 9 8 7 6 5 4 3 2 1

Library and Archives Canada Cataloguing in Publication
Drew, Lorna Ellen, 1937-
Different minds: living with Alzheimer disease / Lorna Drew, Leo C. Ferrari.
ISBN 0-86492-443-7
1. Ferrari, Leo C., 1927- — Health. 2. Alzheimer's disease — Popular works. 3. Alzheimer's disease — Patients — Canada — Biography.
I. Ferrari, Leo C., 1927- II. Title.

RC523.2.D74 2005   362.196'831'0092   C2005-904196-X

Published with the support of the Canada Council for the Arts and the New Brunswick Culture and Sport Secretariat. We acknowledge the financial support of the Government of Canada through the Book Publishing Industry Development Program (BPIDP) for our publishing activities.

Goose Lane Editions
469 King Street
Fredericton, New Brunswick
CANADA E3B 1E5
www.gooselane.com

Dedicated to all those with Alzheimer Disease,
to their caregivers, and especially to Dave,
whose inspiring optimism I will never forget.

By sharing experiences of our uninvited
encounter with Dr. Alzheimer, we can break
through the barriers of silence and loneliness.
Let's not be ashamed of something that is not our
fault. Rather, let us speak out proudly and loudly
about it — even laugh — and realize that while
we last, we too have our contributions to make
to the rich tapestry of human life.

— Leo Ferrari

Grateful Acknowledgements

First and foremost, our thanks to the wonderful women at the Alzheimer Society of New Brunswick, Fredericton: Gloria McIlveen, Chandra Parrot and Leona Gallant. They were, and are, there when we need them.

Pepita Ferrari, who did the first reading of the completed manuscript, for her many helpful suggestions.

Dr. Hazel MacRae, Department of Sociology, Mount Saint Vincent University, who has included Leo's case in her ongoing research on the ravages of Alzheimer disease, *ut scientia progrederetur.*

Our editor, Sabine Campbell, who miraculously fashioned an orderly narrative from shreds and patches.

To the drivers of Fredericton's Checker Cab Company, who always see us safely home.

And lastly, and most gratefully, to our wonderful network of friends, who love us and put up with us, and to whom we turn increasingly for help and comfort.

The Authors Introduce Themselves

A Word from Leo

I am Leo Ferrari, the subject of *Different Minds: Living with Alzheimer Disease*. I was diagnosed with Alzheimer Disease in January of 2003. I decided to write this book since I have always believed that when life gives you lemons, make lemonade.

I was born in Australia in 1927. My first background is in science, and years of practical scientific analysis were followed eventually (in Canada) by years of studying, teaching, and publishing in medieval studies. My first discipline proved to be of enormous advantage in making and clearly explaining new discoveries. I trust that the same will apply to this present task.

After thirty-eight years of teaching, I retired from St. Thomas University and was honoured to be appointed its first Professor Emeritus. So what caused me to become an Alzheimer survivor? Was it all my mental exertions? I hope my story in the following pages will show that there is no connection.

I chose to share my experiences here so that readers may profit from them, especially by recognizing the early signs of the onset of Alzheimer Disease in themselves or loved ones. It is important to recognize these signs for what they really are, because there are medications now available that can be used to slow down the progress of the disease.

A Word from Lorna

When Leo was diagnosed with Alzheimer Disease (AD), he wanted desperately to be able to help others in their struggle with it. To that end, he decided to write a pamphlet sharing his insights. I became involved in the project when I was asked for my input at a joint presentation on the subject. We used a sort of "he said, she said" format, in which I, the caregiver, and Leo, the person living with AD, each presented our individual points of view. Our talk was so popular that we decided to piggyback my text onto Leo's original writing for this book.

Leo has been writing all his life. It's his favourite occupation; working at his desk is the activity he enjoys best. I've never had to worry about whether he was bored or not. A creature of routine, Leo — a scholar who specialized in the writings of St. Augustine — has been totally absorbed in his work for years and years. Most of his time was spent wrestling his theories on St. Augustine into elegant academic articles, though he self-published two books of poetry: *The Worm's Revenge* (1968) and *Over the Edge!* (1977). He calls his pithy little verses "Ferrarigrams."

Alzheimer Disease has robbed Leo of the sustained memory needed to produce lengthy articles, but his language skills continue to provide enjoyment both for himself and others. Out of the proverbial lemons, he continues to manufacture lemonade. As of this writing, he is unable to keep the narrative sequence connecting beginning, middle, and end in his head, so the short, humorous personal essay has become his forte. Many of these essays have been published in the *New Brunswick Reader*, the Saturday supplement of the *Telegraph-Journal*. "It's my new career," he says. "I'm writing funny stories. I love to make people laugh." And laugh they do. People meet him on the street and thank him for the pleasure he's given them.

Leo keeps a list of topics he wants to write about, events that occurred in the past, and he is somehow able to recall enough details to construct three- or four-page stories. Since it is very difficult for him to keep on topic, he writes several drafts, a task he thoroughly enjoys. I sometimes help with the editing, as I did before he had Alzheimer Disease. Still, I am always amazed that he pulls it off.

My background in nursing helped me to be less fearful of the disease, but my writing background, culminating in a PhD in English Literature, proved invaluable. Stories heal, and making narrative sense of a life lived with Alzheimer Disease gives me both the perspective to stand outside events and (sometimes) laugh and the feeling that I have some sort of control over an illness whose symptoms more often than not play havoc with what used to be an ordinary life.

Like Leo, I am glad to do my bit for the cause, to help in the production of the proverbial lemonade, though, as a reluctant caregiver, I find that my preferred metaphor is "biting the bullet." Caregiving, like child-rearing, is all too rife with opportunities for learning on the job. I hope that what I learn as I embark on this new and unforeseen career will be of use to others.

A Primer on Dr. Alzheimer and His Namesake Disease

In 1907, in Frankfurt, Germany, Dr. Alois Alzheimer (1864-1915) published a landmark article about the brain of a "mad" female patient, Frau Auguste D., who had died at the relatively young age of fifty-one. Significantly, her death was preceded by a long period of progressive mental decline and bizarre, noisy behaviour. Later, on examining her brain under a microscope, instead of normal brain cells, Dr. Alzheimer found many varied, tiny abnormalities. They were made all the more conspicuous by the comparative scarcity of normal brain cells.

Alzheimer's theory was that there was direct correspondence between the massive distributions of those various tiny, abnormal cells, and his patient's extremely confused mental condition. Later, the significant presence of similar abnormalities in brain cells was linked to the bizarre behaviour of other patients. Further observations strengthened the connection in the reverse direction; certain kinds of behaviour could predict the abnormalities of the brain cells of such persons.

Alzheimer Disease (or AD), playfully known also as "Old Timer's Disease," is not a normal part of aging, nor is it infectious. It is not a mental illness but a physical disease of the brain, accompanied by various symptoms, the first of which usually is forgetfulness. At 64 % of all the kinds of dementia in our society, AD is certainly the most common one. Among those over sixty-five years of age, 364,000 Canadians (or about one in thirteen) have Alzheimer Disease. People as young as thirty-eight and forty have been diagnosed with it. The disease is about twice as common in women as in men, and women are doubly burdened in that over 70% of informal caregivers are also women, mostly wives or daughters.

The symptoms of AD include, principally, loss of memory, judgement, and reasoning. Changes of mood and behaviour also occur. It is estimated that by the year 2031, the number of Canadians afflicted with AD and related diseases will have doubled from the current 364,000 to over 750,000. Much research is therefore being dedicated to the possible causes of the disease, aimed, of course, at its eventual elimination.

Among the factors favouring (though not causing) AD are advanced age (mostly, though not always, above sixty-five), Down Syndrome, previous traumatic head injuries resulting in unconsciousness, low educational or occupational attainment, gender, Parkinson's Disease, race, certain environmental toxins, bad diet, lack of exercise, and prolonged depression. Doubtless this list will be extended over time.

To tell you about my particular case, I had a traumatic head injury at the age of ten. After "stealing" a ride on the rear of a van, I panicked as it got farther and farther away from home, finally jumping from the speeding vehicle. Not then understanding the laws of motion, I hit the pavement head first. This resulted in three days of unconsciousness and a massive swelling of the bruised area around my right eye. The local newspaper at the time complicated things further by reporting that I had been killed after jumping from my own father's car! Much later in life — also on the negative side where my memory is concerned — I worked with a great variety of toxic chemicals during my first career as an analytical and research chemist. These included cyanides and insecticides, such as DDT and BHC, and a variety of organic solvents. Without further research it is difficult to say how large a role these factors played in my own eventual diagnosis.

The Sneaky Disease

Leo

AD certainly should be called "the Sneaky Disease." Believe me. Take it from one who has been there, and who knows by personal, first-hand experience. Catch a cold and you know it's there in a matter of days. But when you have developed AD you can go for years without even suspecting that you have it inside your head, where it is silently working day and night on the deadly destruction of your mind's precious brain cells with their memories of the past. Science is searching both for the cause and for the means of eliminating this affliction, but so far no magical cure or prevention has been discovered.

The onset is so gradual that it is impossible to identify, but looking back, certain now-significant examples stand out. For instance, in 2002 my wife and I spent a very pleasant evening over supper with two friends. At one stage I recalled the days long before washing machines, when we did all the washing by hand. Then followed my detailed account of boiling the clothes in a large copper vessel, then rinsing them, then "blueing," and wringing them by hand, before hanging them out to dry on the clothesline. The problem was that when my wife remarked on this description the next morning, I had absolutely no memory of having made it. I thought that was really weird at the time, but its significance was only later to dawn on me.

The doubly deceptive nature of AD is that it is painless, as it slowly sneaks up on its unsuspecting victim. As it takes over, AD causes an ongoing series of silent thefts from the Treasury of Memory. While memories of the distant past usually remain solidly established, the theft begins with the recent memories. This can start sometime in middle age (range: forty to sixty years), or (rarely) even sooner. Furthermore, unlike the common cold, it does not come from outside but is internal in origin, from unknown causes, and it results in a slow degeneration of the brain itself.

Since AD develops gradually over years, early detection is urgent for this important reason: thanks to modern medication its progress can be slowed down considerably. With early medication, the person with AD can reach an older age in far better condition than would have otherwise been the case.

In the worst-case scenario, living with advanced Alzheimer Disease will be like living in a fog. At least this was the impression I first had of it. I am reminded of a poem by the poet Hermann Hesse (1877-1962), one I learned long ago when studying German. Here is my translation of the first verse:

> *Strange — wandering in the fog!*
> *Each bush and stone is alone.*
> *No tree sees the other,*
> *Each one is alone.*

Lorna

In retrospect, I think Leo had Alzheimer symptoms several years before he was tested. On a holiday in Mexico in 1999, he was unable to retain any information about where we were going, nor could he recall what luggage he would need.

When we had settled in, to my horror and with disastrous results, he brushed his teeth with tap water, although he'd been repeatedly warned against doing so, and was stricken with a nasty case of diarrhea, fever and vomiting. On several occasions during our stay he was confused. For example, he thought he was back in Australia, and at one point I found him looking for St. Augustine in the refrigerator in our hotel room.

At the time I blamed the tap water, putting his bizarre behaviour down to the high fever and medication, but it really was far worse than you might expect given the circumstances. There was a little church near our apartment, and though I'm not a Catholic, I'd go in every day and ask St. Anne to help me get this man back to Canada. We did get home, and Leo was mentally much better on our return, though the intestinal upset lasted for weeks afterwards.

I now know that, typically, people with AD become much worse when taken out of their routines. I am convinced that Alzheimer Disease was the cause for all Leo's confusion. On another holiday, in 2002, he needed to be constantly oriented as to where he was, why he was there, and who our hosts were. In between trips his absent-mindedness had increased, but it was that holiday abroad in 2002 that made me insist on medical testing.

Leo

At first, like many others, I resisted getting tested for Alzheimer Disease, reciting where necessary my long-range memory achievements. But meanwhile, by day and night, and without my knowledge, let alone consent, my precious Memory Bank was being steadily robbed of its most recent additions. In essence, a famous brainy bank robber was at work (initials: A.D.). Mr. A.D. is the most sneaky and audacious of all robbers, stealing our recent memories before we can file them away in the safer storage areas of the more distant past. Last in, first to go.

Well, there are arguments against getting tested. For example, I may have forgotten what I did yesterday at noon, or what I had for supper last night, but arguably this is mere short-term memory loss. "Just stop bugging me, and I can remember anything I want to!" In line with this position (as I used to argue with Lorna), I still frequently meet people on the street whom I have not seen for years, yet I know their names immediately. Seeing that I have such an excellent long-term ability for remembering, how could I possibly have a genuine short-term memory problem? It's just the pressure of the moment, making me nervous and blocking off my memory (I hoped). But is it possible that my situation is far more serious than I want to admit?

Quite recently, in three separate encounters, my dramatic demonstrations of being able to recall immediately names and details from the distant past were so certain and convincing that I kept refusing to face the dreadful possibility that perhaps I was yet another victim of AD. Above all, I insisted to my nearest and dearest, my ability to recall these names instantly was proof positive and certain against her suspicion that I might be another member of the Alzheimer club.

But I realize at this late date that, had Lorna asked me to draw up an itemized list of what I did yesterday, I would have been incapable of doing it. Had that challenge been issued and accepted, it would have been obvious to both of us that something was drastically wrong with my memory.

Diary

*Brunch with friends. Leo was fine. Knew
who they were, told some old stories, but
didn't repeat himself a lot. He's quieter than
he used to be, and I think it's because he can't
take in information sufficiently quickly to
take part in the conversation, so he listens,
smiles, and waits for a memory trigger. I told
him that I sometimes like him better with
Alzheimer. It's made him unsure, but he has
lost the fierce righteousness he used to have
about so many things.*

The Alibi of the
Absent-Minded Professor

Leo

There are persistent symptoms in favour of getting tested for Alzheimer Disease. The principal sign to look for in yourself or in your partner is an increase in forgetfulness. In this respect, as the recipient of many remarks about my memory, I want to point out how important it is to pay attention to these remarks, rather than to go heavily into defiant denial.

Of course, I had a valuable alibi — I was a professor, and professors are notoriously forgetful, whence the well-known cliché. The "absent-minded professor" usually has his mind on more important affairs than ordinary mundane matters. Indeed, as a professor I liked the adjective absent-minded; it went with the territory. Misreading the signs bolstered my self-image, but at the same time, it allowed AD to destroy more of my precious memory cells. And the destruction would be irreversible!

Basic causes for ordinary absent-mindedness are simple enough. Professors, like a lot of other dedicated professionals, are given to fiercely focusing over a prolonged period of time on some academic problem that intrigues and challenges them. In itself, this concentration and the resulting forgetfulness has nothing at all to do with AD. But AD cannot be automatically excluded.

Being a professor and intensely interested in my specialty, I was typically absent-minded and secretly proud of it. So what was the problem? Well, eventually, at least in my observant wife's opinion, I was absent-minded just a bit too often. At first I hotly denied any accusations. I was just into my early seventies, healthy in diet and daily exercise, and considered myself too young for this "old timer's" illness. I was a most unlikely potential candidate.

Fortunately, my partner was adamant in her insistence on the desirability of having me tested. Finally I had to admit, on the basis of many recent, blatant examples, that perhaps she had a point. With her strong encouragement, and for the sake of family peace, I reluctantly made an appointment to visit our family doctor.

Diary

Went to hear a talk last night with a friend. Over dinner, Leo must have asked twenty times where we were going and who was speaking. My friend said it would drive her nuts to have to live like that. She's right. It's driving me nuts.

The Family Doctor

Leo

The doctor gave me a few tests for Alzheimer Disease. These were all simple (and I do mean really simple) tests, like correctly filling in the numbers on a diagram of a blank clock-face dial, or repeating a recently heard short list of items. Her initial "verdict" was indecisive, and I was told to return at a later date. Some months later, the verdict from a retesting was that there was definitely no evident cause for concern. I returned home with a triumphant feeling of self-righteousness. But as I learned later, my family doctor, unaware of the truly sneaky nature of AD, had examined me for its really advanced stage.

Lorna

Leo actually flunked that first "simple" test in the doctor's office. Although he could draw a clock, he had no idea of the day or month. Our doctor was concerned and retested him three months later. This time Leo, with the wit to memorize the date and month, got an A + and the comment "he's just inattentive" from the doctor.

Around the same time, Leo had hip replacements, and we were told that memory loss could be a result of the anaesthetic. However, I remained concerned. Leo was unable to locate items in our house, items that had been in the same place for years. "Where's the honey?" he would ask, though putting honey on his morning toast was something he'd done throughout all our married life. I would ask him to put away towels, and he couldn't find the linen closet. Moreover, he had no recollection of events of the previous day. Each yesterday was like a blank slate.

Leo

While yesterday, or even this morning, was gone, I could easily recite all sorts of details about my distant past. For example, I can still remember so far back as the time we lived at my maternal grandfather's place at 187 Johnson Street, Annandale, Sydney, Australia. I was only a few years old and slept in a cot with vertical varnished brown slats (each about an inch and a quarter wide) surrounding me on all four sides. My parents slept on a mattress a few feet away. I even remember one morning with the sun streaming down into our basement bedroom, and from the otherwise silent street up above us a man's voice and his horse's hooves going "clop . . . clop . . . clop. . . ." He was calling out, "clothes props . . . clothes props." Later I discovered that these were slender tree trunks about six feet long, used to prop up the washing hung up to dry in our back yard, long before the invention of clothes-drying machines.

Lorna

Leo's problems were definitely much more serious than simple absent-mindedness. We returned to the doctor's office and I asked for a referral to the memory clinic. When, some weeks later, the specialist at the memory clinic said, "You do have Alzheimer, Mr. Ferrari," the die was cast. Although not unexpected, the verdict was still a shock. I had hoped for a diagnosis of non-progressive dementia, if there is such a thing. Not Alzheimer. Not us.

Leo

Our experience brings out a very important aspect of the early recognition of AD — I was the last person capable of judging whether I had it or not. The person most qualified to be the judge in this respect is someone with whom the person with suspected AD comes in prolonged, daily, intimate contact — and in my case that is Lorna, my partner. Those who are not so accompanied just have to wing it, or else try unusually hard to be completely honest with themselves. In any case, my first natural reaction was denial.

No doubt the inability to face the enormity of such a situation is the reason many people who experience "absent-mindedness" can dismiss it as merely a temporary thing. When pushed further, they can even try to explain it away as simply spontaneous resistance to being questioned. Such uninvited intrusion (they claim) blocks the brain's endless ability to recall memories at will. In other words, the interference is making the person nervous, and so prevents him from performing spontaneously, when (hopefully) there is no memory problem at all.

To support this dithering you might use the analogy of "exam fever." This is the traumatic experience of some students who know everything about the test material until they find themselves in the exam room. Then their memory becomes like a blank slate. In a way, it is also like stage fright, when some children have memorized everything, until they get up there on the stage and their minds go absolutely blank. Later, as adults, such people might easily rebel against being examined by a memory specialist, so possibly allowing AD to continue its silent sabotage.

Ferrarigram	*A Laugh*

Mine is a wild voice
Laughing out
In the loneliness
      — from *Over the Edge*

Lorna

Everybody thinks they're exempt from disaster until it happens. We're certainly no exception. We eat well, exercise, involve ourselves in the community, have an active social life and, even in retirement, meaningful work. We recycle and compost. We're good people doing good-people things, and that's the point; research has not yet come up with solid reasons why the numbers of people afflicted with Alzheimer Disease are reaching epidemic proportions (though pollution has been cited). Bad things happen to good and bad people alike.

That said, I confess to an initial tendency to blame the victim. When our family doctor said Leo was "just inattentive," I couldn't have agreed more. Validation at last! I went on repeating the old refrain "you never listen," until I was sick of saying it. But clearly, this went beyond mere inattentiveness, medical authority notwithstanding. The whole thing came to a head when I went out one night and came home late to a desperately worried and irate husband who opened the door with the words, "The police are looking for you." He'd forgotten where I'd gone, and it wasn't the first time. Episodes like these had prompted us to ask for a referral to the memory clinic in the first place.

The Alzheimer Specialist

Leo

Much valuable time was wasted between my first visit to the family doctor and my appointment with an Alzheimer specialist. There, on January 2, 2003, I underwent a series of tests, some of which produced undesirable results. To put it bluntly — I flunked! I was promptly put on daily medication aimed at slowing down the ongoing degeneration of my brain cells. After all — an ounce of prevention is worth a pound of cure. At last I was on the right path and no longer had to struggle with the "NOT ME" syndrome.

My specialist referred me to two other kinds of specialists within a few weeks. First I visited a psychologist at our hospital, and he put me through a new series of tests (all perfectly painless) to find out precisely where my mental strengths and weaknesses lay. Having spent at least an hour at these tests, I returned about a week later (not without some anxiety) to receive the results and the explanations of their significance.

The tests were classified into four categories, and in order of descending grades the results were as follows: first came Reasoning, where I received the grade of "Unusually Good"; next was Math Problems in which I was rated as "Normal"; in Concentration my ranking was "Not Too Bad"; and my weakest result by far was Memory, where I ranked as "Defective," in other words, an F. Me, a professor! But looked at positively, it was the most important F of my life.

You can't always win them all. On the other hand, if there is something wrong, the important thing is to come to terms with it as soon as possible. I was told to report for a repetition of the same tests a year later, to see what changes, if any, had occurred. Meanwhile, I was to live a healthy life, never forgetting to take my pill each night.

But flunking some simple tests was, to me — a scholar — unthinkable. I was still not completely convinced of my new role as someone with AD. Accordingly, I applied for and succeeded in obtaining the second set of tests some six months later, rather than the proposed whole year. The time eventually came around, and I tried my very hardest to get better results. Alas, essentially the same results were obtained. This proved one definite thing: despite my best academic results in the past, willpower and preparation had nothing to do with the results of the tests for AD. On the other hand, the experience did finally make me accept my condition.

Diary

How do other people live on this emotional roller coaster? How do I? I can stand the despair; it's the hope that's driving me mad. Today, after a dinner with friends at our house, Leo, whose back was to the living room, said, "What happened to that piano you used to play?" I told him to turn around, and there, of course, was the piano. My heart drops when these things happen. I get angry because I'm so scared. We'd had wine with dinner, which makes him more confused, and he was tired. Later on, his son called from Montreal, and Leo was able to tell him about details of our lives I didn't think he'd remember. But the dementia is increasing all the same.

Still, some people lose it a lot faster than Leo. The father of a friend of mine went to a nursing home only months after his diagnosis. His first symptom was failure to recognize his wife. He couldn't figure out why the cleaning lady was sleeping with him.

I collect stories like this. Horror stories which are also funny stories. If you're going to be on this ride, your routine might as well include laughter. Listening to other people, and hearing their stories, I feel like I'm a member of a club I hadn't even known was out there.

Leo

My second referral was for a CT scan of my brain. This scan would determine whether there was anything else organically wrong with my brain. I must say I admire the scan's thoroughness. The scanning machine, compared with the size of my head, was monstrous indeed, and I had to lie inside it. For comfort, not knowing what to expect, I secretly thought of it as an oversized X-ray machine, and, much impressed by its size, I braced myself for a jolt that it might perhaps deliver, especially when I was told to keep very still. Imagine my relief when, after I had felt nothing at all, a voice told me I could leave. I even felt somewhat cheated. All that anxiety for nothing!

Lorna

People, in an effort to be helpful, have suggested a variety of remedies purported to cure or arrest AD. In our experience these remedies are not only expensive but useless. Leo and I have used various homeopathic remedies for years, and although useful for many conditions, none has been helpful in alleviating his Alzheimer symptoms (although, who knows, they may have delayed their onset). Acupuncture, aroma therapy, and reiki all claim success in treating a variety of illnesses, but many insurance plans don't cover the cost of these treatments, which, in the case of a chronic illness such as Alzheimer Disease, can be ongoing. Vulnerable people may therefore go through their savings hoping for the cure so far denied them by traditional medical treatments. Vitamins too are expensive and often not covered by a drug plan.

I heard one of the more off-the-wall recommendations at our local market. An acquaintance suggested avocados would help. Unfortunately for our food budget, Leo proceeded to buy them in bulk. Every time I opened the refrigerator door, more avocados would fall out. Because nowhere in the literature on Alzheimer was there any mention of the benefits of avocados (and because I was beginning to suspect that our informant had business interests in Mexico) I put a stop to this profligacy.

One day, and as a further example of how susceptible we had become, I received a call from a woman who had read an article about Leo's struggle with AD in our local paper. She said that she could help him, and suggested we make an appointment with her. I was appalled that anyone would try so shamelessly to take advantage of us. I told her, with finality, that we weren't interested. The episode at least made me aware that we had become targets for snake-oil sellers.

So, I Have AD — Why ME?

Leo

For the last quarter century my partner Lorna and I have
been great patrons of our local health food store, and have,
through their book section, read widely on regular exercise
and diet for promoting good health. Furthermore, the
store's well-read owner ("Doctor Ralph," as I like to call
him) is a living fountain of information on nutrition and
healthy living. I remember a sign that I used to see on my
way to classes at Sydney University every morning: "What
you eat today, walks and talks tomorrow." In other words,
"we are what we eat," and good nourishing food with
plenty of fruit, vegetables and vitamin supplements is
basic to any healthy life. As for diet, it's a poor attitude to
think that just because you like something it must be good
for you.

On the exercise aspect of good health, my dear old
father used to say: "You should get out of breath at least
once a day." I have tried to live this way, day by day, but I
have had to develop strategies, since so much of my life

has been devoted to books and writing. The best place to start was exercise in the form of daily walking to and from school and university. Later in life we were blessed in living close to a pool. First thing in the morning, a vigorous swim is the very best way to set you up for the day.

Some years later we had to move away from any pool, but by advertising in the local paper I was inundated by responses from people who had second-hand exercise bikes for sale. After that, first thing in the morning I jumped on my bike and (while reading a book) pedalled away vigorously for at least fifteen minutes daily. Believe me, once you get addicted, there's no better, faster way to start the day.

More recently, we acquired a lovely little poodle, Barkis. I'd been walking him every day until the light went on and I realized that I could better utilize this activity by alternately jogging (a hundred, then, later, two hundred paces), then walking. Barkis enjoys it as much as I do, and he can run much faster. If you have to take your dog for a walk every day, that's a chore, but if you take him for a daily run — that's exercise! Those who are vigorously inclined can always find a way.

Getting back to the present topic, with a very contented life, a good partner, healthy diet, and regular exercise, why should someone like me come down with AD? Frankly, I don't know. But, stuck with it, the next best thing to do was to see what could be done about it. So the question of the original cause has become irrelevant.

Diary

Had a man over to measure the kitchen floor for linoleum. He met Leo, who, in his usual open way, said, "She handles everything because I have Alzheimer Disease." The two of them had a nice chat, and then the service-man drove me to the warehouse to pick out floor colours. When we were in the car, he said, "My mother had Alzheimer's. You've got such a hard time coming." Oh, that's so frightening. What am I supposed to do now with that information? I wanted to tell him not to say that, not to put that in my face. "And your husband seems like such a nice man," he went on. Oh dear. He was only trying to sympathize. "Yes," I said. "Leo's a lovely man."

The Power of Positive Living

Leo

As I write this, it is over two years since I was first diagnosed. So — I have AD! For many years now I have lived a disciplined life, with a positive attitude, a healthy diet, and regular exercise. Attitude is all-important. If you go through life with a pessimistic outlook, sooner (rather than later) your worst expectations will be realized. If you are optimistic, then fate is loaded in your favour, and I've kept my optimism in the years since I was first diagnosed with AD at the age of seventy-five.

I have always chosen to make lemonade out of life's lemons. Perhaps that is related to the privilege I had of meeting someone in my native Australia well over half a century ago. As long as I live I will not forget him. I met Dave in an old men's "home" while I was doing what we then called "acts of charity," visiting the poor and sick. In reality it was a hospital of wards filled with chronically ill, often bedridden, aged men, who also were the "down and outs" of society. In age, Dave was an exception — he was in his early thirties. He had come from England to participate in a rugby game and unfortunately happened to break his back on the rugby field. In those days any hope of returning to England would have been out of the question.

Week after week, month after month, year after year, there he lay, always on his back, in a ward full of old men. But he did not just lie there. From his pillow he beamed at you, and he always had the best selection of jokes you'd ever heard. Next thing, you'd be splitting your sides with laughter. Beats me where he got the jokes, but he always had a new crop every time I showed up. And it was not just the jokes; it was the joyous way he told them. I have long forgotten Dave's jokes, but I'll never forget Dave. In my later years, hit by the usual blows of life, the memory of Dave and his jokes has always buoyed me up. What a privilege to have known him. Even as I type this, the memory of Dave makes me dewy-eyed. In those depressing surroundings, he radiated the two most valuable, defiant assets of the human condition — happiness and laughter!

In a way, other things being equal, the person with AD is lucky by comparison with Dave. AD will eventually deprive me of the past. There will be the continuing "Fog of Forgetfulness," nothing to laugh or cry about, only the gradual thickening of memory that will eventually envelop me completely. At its worst, in this fog there will be no direction, no past nor future, only the here and now. There is, however, the concern and eventually the grief of my loved ones. May they be granted the bravery of Dave.

Ferrarigram   *Life*

Life's it!
If you can take life
You can take anything.
If you *do* take life
you *do* take anything!
— from *The Worm's Revenge*

Lorna

Following the diagnosis, Leo and I contacted our local Alzheimer association. The help offered us was, and continues to be, invaluable. That's where I met Leona, Gloria and Chandra, the wonderful women who work there; they are *my* caregivers. Leo started going to the group for people with Alzheimer Disease (I don't go because I don't need to yet), and we got all the information we needed to carry on: available medication (Leo received a prescription immediately), theories, research history, what to do if he wanders, legal advice, everything the experts knew about the disease was available to us. We began the process of adjustment by visiting our lawyer. I'm extremely lucky in that Leo was more than willing to have me take control of our finances. I now have power of attorney.

The hard part is, I never wanted monetary control (or any other kind of control, for that matter). Leo's salary was the larger, so we lived on that, and I kept my own earnings. He is the one who has made the investments, kept records, bought insurance, paid for home maintenance, all those "man" things that I was never any good at and was happy to turn over to someone else. He also has a bookkeeping system that I'd never learned anything about. By the time I took charge, the system was a mess, and Leo had forgotten how it worked. Bills came in and he'd forget to pay them. I'd find out when we got a call from the credit card company, wondering where our payment was while they busily racked up interest on the arrears. I don't mean to complain; we'll be all right financially, and I'm okay with managing the money now.

I *have* learned some coping strategies. I watch like a hawk when the mail comes in and appropriate everything to do with money. Everything we have is jointly owned. Leo still has a credit card that he is able to use correctly, but I frisk him when we come home from an outing; otherwise he'll take off his good pants, hide them somewhere, and forget to remove his wallet from the pocket and put it in the designated usual place. We've spent hours looking for his credit card, and still do sometimes, because I'm not always on top of it. And when he misplaces things I get angry. I just can't help it. I get angry because I'm afraid.

Of basic importance to my optimum condition as an AD survivor is "The Problem of the Pill," that is, never forgetting to take it every day. And here's how I do it. Every good pharmacy will be able to sell you a little plastic device that has a compartment for every day of the week (each with a lid that states the day of the week), plus an eighth one. My method is to put the proper pills — one for AD, two for BP (blood pressure) — in each of the seven compartments. In the eighth place I also put the pills — when I get to number eight it reminds me to fill up again for another week. You might ask me how I then remember to actually take the pills. My answer is that I always keep the little box under my pillow, with my pyjamas, so I cannot forget them. The pill-taking is essential since I'm aiming to be around as long as I can, and that requires a method that works.

Another concern of mine was that perhaps my brain needed a good long vacation away from mental activity. However, the psychologist discouraged this. Basically, in a manner of speaking — rest is rust. The important thing to do with one's mind (as well as one's body) is to keep exercising it daily. It is a simple fact that both mentally and physically we are made to move.

Whether you have AD or not, a healthy reaction to the senior years is to choose a hobby, some daily form of mental activity that both stimulates and mentally appeals to you. Some examples are crossword puzzles, cooking, gardening (also inside, if possible), building model castles from used match boxes, knitting, playing checkers, chess, or writing — like I'm doing. Another source of finding interesting pastimes is to visit your local library where you can look up possible hobbies. Anything to exercise the mind and keep it occupied with some enjoyable pastime. The principal desirable considerations are that the occupation be regular, pleasantly active, and mentally challenging. Life — if you don't use it you'll lose it.

Above all, the individual with AD should avoid a mainly passive pastime, such as prolonged sitting and watching TV from sheer boredom. Carried to excess, this combined neglect of both mind and body just dulls the former and undermines the latter, inviting more rapid mental and physical deterioration. Life will become simply not worth living and so ends, not with a bang, but with a prolonged whimper. The challenge of being a healthy Alzheimer club member involves finding both mental and physical means of regular stimulation.

On the other hand, we also need to rest. A good night's sound sleep is of basic importance to the maintenance of good health. As one gets older, sleep can become rather erratic, and some people tend to resort to sleeping pills. Used continually, these can have undesirable side effects. I would rather seek some more natural remedy, like physical exercise during the day, or just before bed, and I've discovered that by exercising last thing at night, I no longer have to get up to pee. Don't ask me why.

The Community

Leo

It is helpful and stimulating to interact with congenial people of about your own age. But as age advances, if you're lucky enough to survive, the built-in penalty is that life can become increasingly a solitary confinement as your friends die off. Here, belonging to a social group for elders can be a kind of lifesaver from loneliness where it will be still possible to foster nourishing friendships with kindred spirits.

The first such community to come to mind is the local Alzheimer Society and its social activities. Another would be church groups, particularly those that cater to seniors. A little inquiring around is the way to investigate this possible resource. Also, in general, groups that are based on common interests are good prospects. The local pub is another possible location, as long as a person has no problem with lack of sobriety. Also, on the basis of personal experience, it is amazing how sustaining social interactions can occur over other liquids, such as tea, coffee, and even mineral water! Sipping and socializing seem to go together.

Lorna

A few weeks ago, I thought it might be easier if we sold our house in the suburbs and moved to a downtown apartment. If Leo (who is registered with the Safely Home Wandering Registry) got lost, he'd be easier to locate. I mentioned this idea to my neighbour. "Why," she asked, "would you want to do that?" I explained. "Don't worry," she said, "we'll look after him." When I thanked her, I had tears in my eyes. We live in a cul-de-sac, a court where we know, and are friends with, all our neighbours. They *will* look after him. In fact, sometimes it seems like the whole of Fredericton knows not only who Leo Ferrari is (partly because of his many years as a popular university teacher, and partly because he's so friendly) but also that he has Alzheimer Disease. Leo has been up front about this from the day he was diagnosed. Cab drivers look out for him. Perfect strangers ask me how he's doing. Living with Alzheimer is much less stressful when the diagnosis is out in the open.

Diary

Leo went out to dinner with his old friend Bob,
something he's been doing once a week for
decades now, so it was with some trepidation
that I answered a call from Bob an hour after
their appointed time. He's asking Leo's
whereabouts. "I don't know" — I'm getting
anxious — "I thought he was with you." We
decide to wait. Half an hour later, Bob calls
again. Still no Leo. Then Bob calls the cab
company and reports that Leo was deposited
in front of the post office, not far from the
restaurant, at five p.m. I contemplate calling
the police, but decide, intuitively, against it.
He hasn't wandered yet. Rather than sitting
home stewing, I call a cab to keep my concert
engagement. Just after depositing me at the
theatre, the cab returns and the driver informs
me that, in response to an all-cars alert, a
driver spotted Leo going into a restaurant
(the wrong restaurant) and asked him to meet
his wife at the Playhouse. At this point I look

up, see Leo, hug him, reroute him to Bob's
house, and go in to the concert, where three
people in the audience, none of whom I know,
ask me how Leo is doing. Our community
cares. I will never lose this man.

The local daily paper is a great source of information about health and about social events. In communities of any size newspapers contain weekly columns with titles like "Activities for Seniors." These contain all kinds of information and notices about stimulating activities and pastimes. Sometimes further information is only a phone call away. The local YMCA is a good place to begin, and societies like the Kinsmen Club, or the Lions Club often have a section specifically for seniors. For seniors who are disabled, the Canadian Red Cross has loan arrangements available for health equipment. Then there are Meals on Wheels, or even Wheels to Meals where food (and sometimes even entertainment) is available externally.

Our town has a Stepping Stones Senior Centre with a monthly schedule of activities. Transportation can be available for special events. Activities include drawing and painting, crafts, writing, group walks, belly dancing, book sales, Tai Chi, group trips here and abroad, plus just plain coffee and conversation at the Centre. Many other towns have the equivalent.

Diary

Leo's grandson Jasper has a birthday coming up. Leo's never been good at keeping track of birthdays. They always take him by surprise. When I reminded him about Jasper's birthday, he called Penticton, wished him a happy birthday, and put a cheque in a card. Then he couldn't find the address and had to abandon the search because we were getting ready to go out, at which point he lost his wallet, found it again, and misplaced his house keys. He must have asked me five times if I had them. When we got home he couldn't find the card. I finally located it and the address and presented it to him, sealed and ready to go. Then he got upset because he couldn't remember if the cheque was in it. I finally persuaded him that it was, because I saw him put it there. We spend a lot of our lives reinventing the wheel.

Leo

I carry my short-term memory in my pocket. My daily pocket diary had frequent references to my early forget-fulness and my acts of self-recrimination. After I was diagnosed, at my observant wife's suggestion, I acquired a larger pocket diary. Soon after, because of my forgetful-ness, I got myself an exercise book, not just for appoint-ments, but also specifically for recording the important details of certain days, details that seemed to slip too quickly and easily into oblivion. After a few years of that, I now buy a thick, one-page-per-day annual diary for the same purpose. Now I can find out what I did yesterday, or even last week, or last month! While I still have incredible powers of long-range memory (as often occurs with people with AD), ask me what I did yesterday and, except for the notes I have written in my pocket diary, I am utterly at a loss for details. However, as genuine as my intent is in main-taining my memory in this way, I first have to remember to refer to the notes for them to fully suit their purpose.

Hopefully (I thought), the daily events would then have a more enduring place in my memory. Leafing through the diary, some of the events do still stand out, but most do not. At least, because of the words of my own inscribed diary, I know that they occurred. Meanwhile, the fog of oblivion has closed in so gradually, so painlessly, that it has to be recognized for what it is. The early symptoms of AD should have forced me to become perfectly honest with my-self long ago. Maybe my story will help someone to succeed earlier in facing up to the enemy, AD, where initially I failed.

Diary

Leo awakes this morning full of ideas for a new project. I used to dread the onset of a project. There was never time for us. Now I'm happy for him. "What is it?" "I'm going," he announces triumphantly, "to write my memoirs." "Well," I say, "that shouldn't take long." And we both laugh.

Leo

Much later, as I am writing this, the problematic "now" still has its share of recent examples of "forgetfulness," but we are learning. For one thing, by mutual agreement we now have a notice board at home. This does not solve all problems, but it helps, though failing to consult and/or notify the notice board is still a concern.

One day recently I prided myself on remembering that our cute little poodle Barkis had not been taken for his daily walk, and I decided to do it right then. The trouble, as my wife patiently informed me, was that not only had she just taken him for a walk a little while before, but she had expressly told me so. Here again that recurring problem. I had absolutely no remembrance of that communication. This kind of performance, starring *moi*, happens often. In this case, however, you can't argue that one partner doesn't listen to the other, when the real cause is AD.

Diary

*The night before we leave to visit my mother
in Kingston, I list off the articles to be packed,
one at a time. Leo puts an item in his luggage,
and I check it on the packing list. The fun
begins after we get it all in there. He's made
his list and is checking it twice. "Where's my
bathing suit?" I tell him it's in there because
the check mark on the list says it is, and please
don't go through the luggage looking for it. I
have established a little oasis of order and
want to keep it. Leo, thwarted, gets on the
computer and e-mails his friends that he's
leaving town. Twice. Then he tells me that the
computer is broken because he's forgotten how
to send the messages. I send them, none too
patiently because it's late, and we finally get
to bed. The plane leaves at six-thirty a.m.
and the alarm goes off at four. "Where's my
toothbrush?" "I need pens." "These aren't
my glasses." Well, I admit that last was
confusing. I'd put his glasses into my spare*

glasses case, since he'd lost his. Eventually
we get on the plane. Around seven-thirty a.m.,
somewhere in the air between Fredericton
and Montreal, he says "Where are we? I'd like
some supper." The confusion relating to the
change of routine is well under way.

Leo

For most people a conversation is usually a pleasant, almost effortless verbal interaction, with fairly spontaneous give-and-take bouncing back and forth and equal interaction between the two participants (somewhat like playing tennis). A while ago, it struck me that the case was quite otherwise, as experienced internally by an Alzheimer survivor (as I refer to myself, so far!), who carries the burden of trying to act an expected part in a conversation, but without a memory script. Cues become extremely important. I was so struck by this revelation that immediately after a very recent dialogue between Lorna and me, I quickly reconstructed it for purposes of illustration. In the following interaction, my *thoughts* are *italicized*, and the **scary** parts are **bold:**

"What did you do this morning?" she asks innocently.
Panic! How do I cope with this big, shapeless clump of words? I play for time, trying to get a grasp on the clump. But

what can I grab onto? Ah! Thank God! She happens to look at my hair with an approving expression. Hmm. *Yes! By George, I've got it!*

"**I got a haircut!**" I blurt out.

"It's neat. I like it. **Where did you get it?**" she asks so casually.

Quick! Think! Quick!

"**Er — in a barbershop,**" I respond hopefully.

"**Which one?**" she asks with innocent curiosity, but still sounding like an inquisitor.

Quick! Think! Think! Yes! The list! I had a list in my top shirt pocket! So — the shopping mall!

"In the shopping mall, yes."

Great! But, what next?

"**And?**" she says expectantly.

Shopping mall? Shopping mall . . . Yes! The list! I must still have the list. I hope! I reach into my top shirt pocket. Relief! At last I have something concrete to go by!

With a big, inner, silent sigh, I read out aloud all the items on the list. All purchased, present and correct.

Whew! I'm home and dry! At least for now.

Diary

His struggle is often so poignant! Today he said, "It's nice meeting new people. I don't feel that I make so many mistakes."

Life for "Alzheimer Survivors"

Leo

The person most immediately involved, of course, is the one who has been diagnosed with AD. And that's me. First, I have the problem of what I call mental digestion, which involves an understanding of the nature of the disease itself and of its progress. Of prime importance in this regard is the literature available at your local Alzheimer society (see Contact Information, page 107).

The more difficult problem is the emotional digestion. This means coming to terms, in my own heart and in the heart of my nearest and dearest, with the diagnosis of AD and all that it involves and will involve in the future.

Those who have to live with someone who has Alzheimer Disease also need information, and this, too, is available from your local Alzheimer society. But, as valuable as it is, information can only take you so far. You may well need to consult a professional counsellor or spiritual adviser.

It would be a drastic oversimplification to see Alzheimer Disease as affecting only one or even two persons. The diagnosis has repercussions on your circle of friends. Here we have the now familiar problem (in another context) of "coming out." There might be some rude shocks. Some friendships could perish because the other person just does not come around anymore, maybe because of an irrational fear of "catching" the disease, and perhaps such a person should seek some professional advice, but that would not be your problem.

Ferrarigram   *Nostalgia*
I used to be nostalgic
As I looked up the slope
Of sunny afternoon
With the trees and houses
And their long shadows
Reaching down at me

But now it's night-time
And I wish I could see
Those shadows again
— from *Over the Edge!*

Lorna

Leo refers to himself as an Alzheimer "survivor." I prefer to reserve that term for the caregivers. Alzheimer Disease, unlike many other illnesses, takes no prisoners. All you can do is live with it. However, life does go on, and living with someone who has the disease has certainly been a learning process, not least because, with caregiving, my faults are in my face. I didn't realize I was so short-tempered. That realization has taught me something, and I am in the process not only of trying to learn patience, but of forgiving myself when I fail.

Interestingly enough Leo's AD has actually produced the odd benefit. He has forgotten what he doesn't like. I am now able to serve food that he would, in happier times, have refused to eat. His inability to locate things in our house, including the liquor cabinet, has becomes a family joke. And I, who consider myself technologically challenged, am now the expert on computer problems.

Furthermore, because we ourselves are open about our situation, people warm to us. I've been amazed at and have learned from the struggles of others. I had no idea so many people coped, with apparent grace, with problems so similar to ours. This sharing of stories has been inspirational. So, indeed, has been our writing this book together; may it encourage others in telling their own stories.

Diary

Today I lost my temper with Leo again. I was
telling him that I'd been making soup for a
fundraiser all day and, after supper, would
have to go back to help put it into containers.
A few minutes later, I told him I was leaving.
"What for?" "I'm going to help put the soup
in containers, remember?" (Remember is the
wrong word to use when you're talking to
someone with Alzheimer, but I don't remember
to stop myself in time.) He looks puzzled.
"Soup?" he says, and I start. "Haven't you
been listening at all? Have you not got a
context for the word 'soup'?" He doesn't. But
he remembered every detail of his walk with
the dog, including how many paces they took.
How come he can't remember what his own
wife has to say? I lost it. "You've never paid
any attention to my interests. What's the
point in having a conversation at all?" "I'll
tape it," he says. That stops me. "You'll
what?" "I'll tape our conversations and then

I can play them back and know what we
said." Now the logistics of this are insane.
We're going to have a tape recorder handy
whenever we talk to each other? But I didn't
even think that was funny, that's how far gone
I was. Now I think it's funny, and dear and
sad too. He was trying to make it right. Now,
of course, he's forgotten all about it.

Leo

I wanted to tell my story of my unwanted encounter with Dr. Alzheimer's Disease so that the readers of *Different Minds* can give fresh thought to repeated episodes of "absent-mindedness." To forget something once in a while is normal, but to forget things frequently could very well be a symptom of Alzheimer Disease.

Its silent, subtle, and painless assault on the victim's brain should not be dismissed, as some family doctors may have done, as "natural forgetfulness." The spouse, relative, or friend who suspects that someone has become too absent-minded should suggest honestly (and courageously) that this person see his or her family doctor and insist on being tested by a professional AD specialist.

Ferrarigram   *Parable of the Ploughman*

> He who puts his hand to the plough
> And turns back —
> Must have forgotten something
>   — from *Over the Edge!*

As I've said earlier, Alzheimer Disease cannot be cured, but its progression can be slowed down considerably by using the appropriate medication, and the person with AD may reach a good age in far better condition. As to the costs of AD, with what can be well argued is the best health care system in the world, most provinces of Canada cover Alzheimer survivors for both medication and hospitalization.

Neither people with AD nor their caregivers should feel isolated or inferior. Local Alzheimer societies have much down-to-earth advice as well as literature on living with AD, and the regular support group meetings provide an opportunity of getting to know others who are going through the ups and downs of Alzheimer Disease. The Alzheimer meetings in my community also provide quite a delicious lunch!

Our local Alzheimer Society offers support to caregivers as well. Regular caregiver gatherings provide not only genuine sympathy but also the sharing of experiences. These meetings offer an opportunity for talking with others in the same situations, sharing concerns, fears and problems, getting first-hand advice. It seems to me that this is the situation for women (who mostly make up the caregivers), but men, who from their earliest years are often burdened with the handicap of having to be "strong," have trouble with expressing their deepest fears and insecurities. This certainly holds true when it comes to talking about their own or their partner's Alzheimer Disease. Personal fears are taboo. As a result, these unexpressed fears build up as silent but consuming parasites, isolating them and preventing the men from getting the relief that comes with sharing worries and fears.

Since my diagnosis with AD I have learned to be frank about it. The bare-naked truth is that there is *nothing* to hide. At first it was incredible, but hard things take time to be *fully* accepted. There is also a natural tendency to save face by keeping silent about some unfortunate things that happen to us. We want to conceal them; yet once we accept the truth, what is there to hide? We are indeed free.

Diary

When Leo remembers things, I rejoice. Even though I know his diagnosis is firm and fixed, there's this little part of me saying, "Well, maybe he doesn't really have it." So when he does something that's clearly right out of the handbook of Alzheimer symptoms . . . I get frustrated and angry at him.

Confessions of a Reluctant Caregiver

Lorna

I never thought I'd be writing and speaking on caregiving, even though I was a registered nurse for many years. (I now refer to myself as a recovering nurse.) The choice of caregiving as a profession wasn't mine; I inherited it because of my sex and class. For middle class girls growing up in the 1950s, whose parents couldn't afford to send them to university yet who wanted their daughters to be able to support themselves if anything went wrong in the marriage (the most important career), there were two options: teaching and nursing. I want you to know that I didn't become an RN because I was keen to save lives and stamp out disease. I chose nursing as a profession because I *really* didn't want to be a teacher. I didn't dislike nursing, but it wouldn't have been my first career pick had other choices been available. Nursing, for me, was a job I did well enough, but I'm not a born caregiver, which is also the reason I chose not to have children. This is what I say to audiences when I speak on caring for someone with AD.

There's a myth out there that says if you're a woman, you're genetically programmed to look after people. It's not true. I was jumpstarted into being a caregiver because my husband has Alzheimer Disease. I didn't ask for this, I don't want it, and I don't like it. Whether or not I love my husband, and I do, is beside the point. I look after him because I'm his wife, and I can, but taking up caregiving again is not what I had in mind for my declining years.

And it's not as though I do it full time — yet. I'm nothing like an expert at this. Leo was diagnosed in January 2003 (he's somewhere in the middle stages now), though I now am sure he had the disease at least five years before that. His forgetfulness had shown up on our trip to Mexico in 1999, starting even before we left home.

Years passed. I noticed that when Leo and I went to a movie, he couldn't recall the plot. For example, he found *The Lord of the Rings*, a movie that children enjoy, confusing. For years, I'd read novels to him, and now he couldn't keep the story straight. Three years of increasing forgetfulness later, and especially when he began asking me where things were located in the house, things that he used on a daily basis, I asked that our family doctor refer him to the memory clinic in Fredericton. When the specialist said, "Mr. Ferrari, you *do* have Alzheimer's," I wasn't surprised, but I was stunned, though Leo wasn't; he wisely said, "Well, we might as well have lunch." But I thought, "Oh God, what do we do now!"

And I started to look long and hard at what the rest of our life might be like, and I say *I* advisedly, because Leo isn't really aware of what's happening. He gets impatient with himself for forgetting, but then he forgets about it. It's not that he doesn't care; he just doesn't realize the enormity of the situation, which is a good thing on the whole. But it does mean that, as his caregiver, I am alone with my emotions about this disease they call the long goodbye. Alzheimer is not a disease where you and the person afflicted can share the emotional burden. It means that you cry by yourself. And here I'm thinking not so much about caring for someone with Alzheimer as I am about the emotions, especially anger and fear, because these are problems for me, the caregiver.

So first I cried, and then I shared our troubles with friends, and I started a journal, parts of which you have already read.

Diary

Things could be worse, he still knows enough not to put the cordless phone in the refrigerator, for example, but he continually starts something, leaves the task incomplete and starts something else. He keeps a daily diary, but it's never handy when he wants to write some-thing down. Or he'll come in from outside, leave his boots on the landing, his coat in the living room, his gloves on the kitchen chair and his hat in the bedroom. At least I always know which way he went. Last week, in twenty below weather, he lost his long johns. He was putting them in the laundry, he said, and got distracted, and they disappeared. They still haven't turned up, along with the 8" x 8" Pyrex baking dish he washed for me not long ago. It's like living with a poltergeist, one of those mischievous little ghosts that appears just to plague you. When the dog needs to go out, the leash is missing. I bought a spare and hid it from Leo. I'm going to need to replace the long underwear and the baking dish too. This replacing of lost objects gets expensive.

Poltergeists and Storytellers

Lorna

One of the hardest things for me to cope with is not being able to find anything. It's the nurse in me. The slogan in the hospital was "a place for everything and everything in its place." If I know where things are, I have control, and knowing that this is an illusion doesn't stop me from enjoying it. So when I can't find things (especially when money's involved, like Leo losing his wallet) I'm a wreck. We spend so much time looking for stuff.

I may be off the wall with this one, but I don't think people who've been married for years and years are necessarily madly in love. I love Leo, but I don't want to be with him all the time and never have. We have very different interests, for one thing. If I want to go to a movie or a play or a talk, he's not necessarily the person I'd choose to accompany me. I have a number of friends and would often prefer to be with them rather than with my husband, who, after all, is not a big fan of shopping or popular culture or modern dance or drama, to mention some of our areas of difference.

Diary

"Learn to live," says one friend, "with mess. Don't expect anything to be where you put it. Expect things to go wrong. Then you can let go of your agenda and enjoy him."

Leo is a storyteller. He has a collection of tales with which he loves to make people laugh, and they do laugh. He's a good storyteller. But I've heard the stories. I can recite them by heart. I don't want to hear them any more. Ever.

Alzheimer Disease means that Leo relates his supply of stories incessantly, whenever we're with people. Now I *do* have ways of getting around this. I can tell him that he's just told that story and doesn't need to tell it again. He's okay with that. But I also realize that stories are his way of engaging socially. He'll wait for a break in a conversation and interject a story. It makes him feel that he's part of the group, and friends and acquaintances certainly don't care if he repeats himself. But I find that very difficult, especially if we're with people I'm really interested in talking with myself. There are no coping strategies for this one. I just bite my tongue.

Diary

*The Buddhists have ways for dealing with
destructive emotions. Lean into them. Don't
try to make them go away. Identify the energy
in the emotion and use it positively. It is, after
all, only energy. It has no substance. Today I
try this and it works. I could feel the anger
rising in my belly. I took a deep breath and
said, "I don't want to explain it again," which
Leo always accepts, except that usually I feel
guilty and explain it again anyway, which
makes me even madder, especially, and
eventually, at myself. After all, how big a
deal is it to explain things again? It's not as
though I have to diaper, wash, and feed Leo.
All I have to do is repeat information.
How hard is that? But it is hard, and I
acknowledge that. It may not be hard for
someone else, and certainly other people
don't mind repeating things to him, but I do.
And it's okay to be me. Today I listened to a
program on Stephen Sondheim and burst into*

tears when they played "Send in the Clowns."
It's my favourite song. "Just when I stop
opening doors / Finally knowing the one that
I wanted was yours / Making my entrance
again, with my usual flair / Sure of my lines /
No one is there." So sad, so beautiful, so
appropriate. Send in the clowns.

Lorna

I've never had children, because I could never imagine what you'd do with them twenty-four hours a day. Right now my life is a whole lot easier than it's going to be. I'm out much of the day, most weekdays, and Leo is in his office, where he wants to be. I'm enjoying life as much as I can, on a one-day-at-a-time basis, including the time we spend together. I read to him. We go to movies, for walks. But we can't have conversations based on shared experiences. There's no longer a pool of shared memories with which to reminisce, events of the day to mull over, opinions, observations to share. Mealtime conversation in our house is pretty well limited to the weather, comments on the food, and what Leo and the dog did on their walk. I'm auditing some university courses, but we can't talk about that. Attempts at conversation about what I'm doing go something like this:

Me: We were talking about poverty in class today.
Leo: Oh? What course are you taking?
Me: Political Science.
Leo: Who's teaching it?
Me: Dr. Bedford.
Leo: How many in the class?

He asks me this every single time I go out the door to class. By the time I've filled in those gaps again, I'm so mad I just don't want to talk any more. So when my friend suggests that I'll enjoy Leo more if I don't worry about a mess, she's right. It will be easier on me. On the other hand, there's not a lot of Leo to enjoy anymore, certainly in terms of talking with him.

Ferrarigram   *Who Am I?*

I —
Who am I?
I am everywhere I've ever been
And all the things that I have seen
And everyone I've ever known.
Yet sometimes when I'm all alone
I ask myself —
Who am
I?

— from *The Worm's Revenge*

Diary

I practice meditation, and I find that it gives me some emotional control. Prayer probably works too, anything that gets your mind off your troubles and gives you some quiet time. Meditation makes me aware of what I'm thinking and feeling when I'm in the thick of it with Leo. The reason this is useful is that I'm not getting feedback from him when I'm in a bad temper. He doesn't validate me. Leo and I used to fight tooth and nail, often at the top of our lungs, then we'd cool off, and then we'd talk. But now I'm the only one who's fighting, who's invested in the argument. He forgets what it's about. Leo's reduced ability to take in information means that my own angry words, missing their target, echo back to me. When you're shouting at someone and not getting any response, it's like looking in a mirror. I can see myself behaving in a way I don't like at all, purple in the face, eyes bulging, thoroughly off-balance, and nobody's fighting with me. When we fight now, most of the time he just looks at me and says, "I'm sorry." It makes me feel like such a shrew.

A couple of days ago I was talking with a friend who'd been a caregiver for years. She has a strategy that I'm going to try next time I need it. "Walk away," she said. "Go into the bathroom and talk yourself down in the mirror. Tell yourself you're okay, you're not a horrible person." "Really?" I said. "Even if my eyes are bulging and my face is purple I'm still okay?" "Yes," she said, "you are."

Me — a Shrew?
Or, Funny, You Don't Look Shrewish

Lorna

In the years before his diagnosis, Leo didn't listen well much of the time, and partly I'm reacting to the old days when I could justifiably say, "You're not *listening* to me!" (I have many friends who say I'm not alone. They claim it's a guy thing.) Now, of course, no matter how hard he listens, he can't process the new information. The situation is radically different, but the old reactions kick in. I think that's why it's good for both of us to socialize. Boredom is something that doesn't get discussed much in relation to living with Alzheimer Disease, but for me it's a problem. I love exchanging ideas and experiences, and thank God I've always had close friends with whom I can do that. I get so *impatient* when Leo doesn't understand what I'm talking about. Why is it so much easier to be patient with other people?

Diary

I think I've figured out why this is so. Other people go away. However irritating, they will eventually go away and leave you alone. The person with whom you live hangs around and irritates you all over again. When Leo irritates me, my insides feel heavy which causes me to snap at him. When I lighten up, I tell him I'm sorry. And then it happens all over again. And again. It's Chinese water torture, is what it is. Drip, drip, drip. By the end of some days I'm positively soggy, hung over with these sensations I wish I didn't own.

I'll tell you something though. When you're on an emotional roller coaster, you know you're alive. I pay attention to how I'm feeling much more than I ever used to. It matters now. This is something that's not going to go away. Leo's attempts to make sense of an ever-receding world are sometimes so poignant they stop me in my tracks. It's why I started keeping a journal, in fact. I wanted to remember specific times, both good and bad.

I don't want to sound as though life is totally burdensome now. In many ways, Leo shares in our household activities. He walks the dog, washes the dishes, makes the bed, changes the sheets, goes out with his own male friends, and remembers to take his medication. Things are going to get a lot worse, but right now we're doing okay. I do want to note the small stuff before times get really tough. I need to know my levels of tolerance, to know what I can do and know what's important. The idea of becoming a full-time caregiver, unable to leave the house even for a moment is, for me, appalling. But I have a network of friends who have offered to help, and the Alzheimer Society will tell me how to access the resources I need to give myself a break. I can't do this alone.

Diary

*When I get home from class today, Leo is excited. He has something new to tell. He wants me to know that when he took the dog out, he inadvertently let two possums onto the back porch. "I shooed one out," he said, "but the other one got away, and I couldn't find it. It's still there somewhere." Possums? Are there possums in Canada? This is not boring. I'm not even sure what a possum looks like. I'm surprised that Leo does. Then the light dawns. "Leo," I ask carefully, "can you describe a squirrel?" He closes his eyes, thinking. "It's small," he says, "and fluffy." "Does it have a tail?" "No," he says, "squirrels don't have much of a tail," and I'm left wondering what the **hell** is on the back deck. It's got to be a squirrel, but what if it isn't? I don't think I really want to know.*

Diary

"I Will Never Leave You"

Today I go to speak at a meeting with student nurses and caregivers at the Alzheimer Society. The students are doing a community project, putting together a pamphlet about the transition of people with dementia (including Alzheimer) from home to nursing home. Almost immediately I learn a new word. I learn that most people in nursing homes are dementing. "Dementing?" I ask, startled. "Is that what you call it?" And yes, it is.

"They," those nursing home inhabitants, are, in one way or another, dementing, and why not? New words are necessary to define the epidemic this disease has become. And anyway, I think I'm more invested in the word "they." This is Leo we're talking about, my husband, not one of "them," a cipher in the system. I'm not used to thinking of him in terms of who he may/will become, an inmate in a nursing home, dementing. I want to go home.

Another caregiver (and, I realize, I too am part of a "them") is afraid. She doesn't want to think about what will become of her husband. I recognize myself six months earlier and feel bonded and, somehow, more comfortable. We are together in this. We will speak of this thing that will happen, and we will do what we can. The nurses want to know how our respective partners are reacting to the inevitability of life in a nursing home. As it turns out, we don't know, because "they" never bring it up. I remember telling Leo, shortly after his diagnosis, that recourse to a nursing home might be necessary. He said he'd prefer that to being a burden. But I don't think he realized, as I did, the enormity of the situation. No more repetitions, no more repeating myself, no more listening to his stories, no more Leo, whom I love. I told the group that I would bring it up with him *again and let them know his reaction.*

At home, when I speak to him of this, tears come to his eyes. "Leo," I say, hugging him, "don't leave me." He returns my hug. "I will never leave you," he says, "even when I die," but his eyes are cloudy with the disease, and he's not really thinking about it. Nor am I. I will take this encounter to the nursing students. They, as they should be, are concerned with the patient. But when the time comes, the patient will have nothing identifiable as choice. These things, the "wheres" and "whens" of nursing home care, devolve upon the caregiver, as do the financial arrangements, funeral options, living wills, life and death choices that I had assumed would be made together.

Later, I tell a friend about that meeting in detail. She praises my courage, what she understands as my ability to detach myself and articulate lucidly what must be emotionally so difficult to bear. "I couldn't do this," she says, and I want to bite her, want to yell at her that yes, she could, and anyway it hasn't happened yet, and I don't know how it will be.

Two caregivers at the meeting had just admitted their partners to nursing homes. They were articulate too. Does this mean that there were no tears, no grief? And of course my friend could do this. The world is full of people who can do this, and who do it because it has to be done. I am no braver than anyone else. As a Buddhist I know that life is about suffering, loss, and death, and I meditate on these things. That doesn't mean I'm detached. Oh, really, it does not mean that. "The drugs help," I joke, and because I've known her a long time, and we are friends, I remind her of the suffering in her own life, and of her courage. She doesn't believe me, doesn't want to talk about it. "It's a beautiful day," she says, and we both laugh.

Safely Home

Lorna

Because many Alzheimer sufferers tend to wander, the Wandering Registry, as it was originally called, was started in a few locations in Canada as a partnership between Alzheimer societies and the RCMP. Thanks to the initiative of the Alzheimer Society in Fredericton, the service, now called "Safely Home," is available across Canada. Registration costs $25. The person with the disease receives a bracelet with a registration number, name, city, and the message, "MEMORY LOSS, CALL POLICE." The caregiver also provides the local police department with a recent photograph. Caregivers can obtain information and registration forms from their local Alzheimer Society. In the United States, this program is called "Safe Return."

Recently, Leo and I travelled to a convention in Wolfville. While I was attending a workshop, Leo and a friend explored the town and went out to dinner, after which the friend returned Leo to the home where we were billeted, sat him down in the living room, told him I'd return soon, and left for his own motel. Leo, apparently not at all confused, complied. Around ten-thirty that night, after the workshop ended, friends and I returned to the house. Leo was not there. I didn't panic; he'd never wandered before and I simply assumed that he was with our friend. Half an hour later, I called the motel. "I left him," said Robert, "at the house."

On one side of the house was the highway, on the other, woods. I called the police. "We've been trying to get you," they said. "He said you'd call." Leo, realizing he was in a strange place in strange surroundings, had assumed that he was lost, walked in the dark to the nearest neighbour, knocked on the door, and told them he had Alzheimer Disease and couldn't find his wife in that weird house across the street. They saw his bracelet and called the police.

It was my first experience with wandering, and it was terrifying. From this time forward, I will make sure that the person caring for Leo never, ever leaves him alone. Leo talks a perfectly lucid game. He will promise what he can't deliver. Although he may show no apparent signs of confusion, out of his element he is no longer operating on all cylinders.

The fact that Leo will happily explain to strangers that he has Alzheimer Disease and needs help is such a bonus. And to my credit, I had registered him with Safely Home. Though I didn't think so at the time, we did well. Both of us.

Diary

Leo and I are packing to go to a cottage for a week. We don't need much. I make out the packing list and we bring the luggage up from the basement. This should be simple. Low stress. Easy. It's not. I hear Leo on the phone saying, "We'll be gone for two weeks." This is not true, and I ask him to hang up. He was, as it turns out, leaving a message with the Alzheimer Society. I explain that I have already done this. I have also cancelled the papers and alerted the neighbours and a number of friends. At my request, he stops reinventing the wheel. We begin the packing dance. Bathing suit. Check. Two shirts. Check. Socks. Check. All is in order, except that his copy of the manuscript for the Alzheimer Society we've been working on is missing, and so is the dog. We return to the basement and locate the papers on his chaotic desk top. A pathetic whine issues from the storage cupboard. Oh good, the dog has turned up

too. I go to my office and start my packing.
Leo appears in the doorway. "I can't find
my bathing suit." I explain about the packing
list. He goes away and I hear him calling the
Alzheimer Society. It's going to be a long day.

Lorna's Tips for Caregivers

Learn to anticipate what can go wrong.
I've taken to frisking Leo for wallet and keys whenever we return from activities outside the home. If I don't, he'll change his clothes, forgetting that these items are in the pockets of the ones he's just discarded.

Never start a sentence with "Do you remember . . . ?"
Conversations begun with those words are doomed to failure. He doesn't remember, but he will spend a lot of effort trying and feel badly when he fails.

When going on a trip, make packing checklists.

Ask friends and family not to leave telephone messages with Leo.
Leo faithfully writes down messages, but he transcribes them on bits and scraps of paper which, most of the time, I find, but which sometimes turn up days later. Friends now know enough to call back if they haven't received a

response from me after a reasonable amount of time. Inevitably, I suppose, I'll need to have recourse to a cell phone.

Spend time looking at photo albums of our travels.
It's a stress-free way of connecting with the past that we can both enjoy. And I cherish the times when he looks at a snapshot and says, "Oh, I remember that."

Be appreciative of what your loved one can do.
I'm amazed at Leo's ability to fix appliances. He also does a lot of household work, including making beds, doing dishes, washing clothes, taking out the garbage and walking the dog. I notice that I'm a lot busier when he's not there. I stopped letting him put groceries away because I can't find some of them. But he wants so much to help and is so proud when he does. Someone asked me, "Why don't you let him? What else are you doing?" Well, yes. How long does it take me to locate a couple of missing items anyway?

Never assume that something that you have asked your loved one to do is done.
When I ask Leo to do something, he needs to do it immediately, otherwise he forgets. I used to get really angry when, hours later, I'd find his clothes still scattered throughout the house, or the heat not turned down. Now I either wait until he's free to fulfill a request before I ask, or I repeat it.

Get power of attorney.

Leo had no trouble with this whatsoever. Shortly after he was diagnosed, we went together to our lawyer's office, where we signed a document giving decision-making power to me. Relevant business and financial institutions now have copies. I continue, however, to keep Leo informed and ask for his opinion on any decisions I need to make affecting us both. Leo, a child of the depression, was always anxious about money matters. I, on the other hand, was a wild and somewhat reckless spender. Now that I have power of the purse, I find myself as anxious about spending as he used to be (which doesn't mean that I don't spend, it's just that I worry about it).

Try to have mail addressed to the caregiver.

What happens in our house is that, if Leo gets his hands on incoming mail and removes it to his basement office, chances are neither one of us will ever see it again. This has, unfortunately, resulted in our having to pay some hefty interest charges. I've since asked companies to address letters to me. Leo, to his credit, now only opens personal letters

Till Death Us Do Part

Lorna

A major concern now is the possibility of nursing home care for Leo in the final stages of the disease. I hope I can keep him with me until death do us part, but given my high level of impatience, I fear that psychologically I won't last the distance, to say nothing of how it would affect me physically. If I can't — as the New Brunswick law stands now — the nursing home will take half of everything we own, with the exception of our house, and by that time we may not be able to afford the upkeep. There's really no way to plan for this contingency. We might as well start spending now, because that rainy day we were saving for has arrived. Furthermore, nursing home fees are levied based on a couple's joint income three years previous to application for care. It seems churlish to complain, because we're probably better off financially than many people. I really just have to hope we can manage. Leo is sensitive to the possibility of nursing home care. He decidedly doesn't want to be a burden, and wants me to do what's best for me. This is hard. I had hoped together we'd both be making decisions about where to live when we're old.

Diary

I'm auditing a course in philosophy and, for my sins, reading Aristotle's Politics. *At one time I would have been able to share my enthusiasm with my philosopher husband. Not now. I am deeply impressed with the ancient Greek's concern for living well, for how to live the good life. What question is more important than that? I look up from the page at my own life. Through the window, October light shines golden off the poplar tree, patterning the walls with light and shadow. There are yellow chrysanthemums on the dining room table, a Berber rug on the polished wood floor. The room is full of art and light. One of Leo's paintings hangs on the wall, a bird flying over the desert, a symbol of hope and regeneration. He hasn't painted in years, but he used to be good. The rocking chair cushions our little poodle. This is the good life. We've been so lucky. We still are.*

Contact Information

Alzheimer Societies

Your local Alzheimer Society has information on the programs and services available in your area. Here you will find invaluable information sheets, books, and videos to help guide you through the Alzheimer journey. You will also find individuals who understand what you are going through and will support you in any way they can.

Below are the regular mail and e-mail addresses, toll free phone numbers, and web sites of the Alzheimer Society of Canada and the provincial offices, and the head office of the Alzheimer's Association in the United States.

Alzheimer Society of Canada
20 Eglinton Avenue West, Suite 1200
Toronto, ON   M4R 1K8
Phone: (416) 488-8772   Toll free: 1-800-616-8816
Fax: (416) 488-3778
E-mail: info@alzheimer.ca
Web site: www.alzheimer.ca

Alzheimer Society of Alberta and Northwest Territories
10531 Kingsway Avenue
Edmonton, AB   T5H 4K1
Phone: (780) 488-2266   Toll free: 1-888-233-0332
Fax: (780) 488-3055
E-mail: edmonton@alzheimer.ab.ca
Web site: www.alzheimer.ab.ca

Alzheimer Society of British Columbia
#300 – 828 West 8th Avenue
Vancouver, BC   V5Z 1E2
Phone: (604) 681-6530   Toll free: 1-800-667-3742
Fax: (604) 669-6907
E-mail: info@alzheimerbc.org
Web site: www.alzheimerbc.org
BC Dementia Helpline: 1-800-936-6033

Alzheimer Society of Manitoba
120 Donald Street, Unit 10, Mezzanine
Winnipeg, MB   R3C 4G2
Phone: (204) 943-6622   Toll free: 1-800-378-6699
Fax: (204) 942-5408
E-mail: alzmb@alzheimer.mb.ca
Web site: www.alzheimer.mb.ca

Alzheimer Society of New Brunswick
33 Main Street,
Fredericton, NB   E3A 1B7
Phone: (506) 459-4280   Toll free: 1-800-664-8411
Fax: (506) 452-0313
E-mail: info@alzheimernb.ca
Web site: www.alzheimernb.ca

Alzheimer Society of Newfoundland and Labrador, Inc.
687 Water Street, PO Box 37013
St. John's, NF A1E 1C2
Phone: (709) 576-0608   Toll free: 1-877-776-0608
Fax: (709) 576-0798
E-mail: sharing@avalon.nf.ca
Web site: www.alzheimer.ca/english/offices/provinces/nf.htm

Alzheimer Society of Nova Scotia
5954 Spring Garden Road
Halifax, NS   B3H 1Y7
Phone: (902) 422-7961   Toll free: 1-800-611-6345
Fax: (902) 422-7971
E-mail: info@alzheimer.ns.ca
Web site: www.alzheimer.ns.ca

Alzheimer Society of Ontario
1200 Bay Street, Suite 202
Toronto, ON   M5R 2A5
Phone: (416) 967-5900
Fax: (416) 967-3826
E-mail: staff@alzheimeront.org
Web site: www.alzheimerontario.org

Alzheimer Society of Prince Edward Island
166 Fitzroy Street
Charlottetown, PE   C1A 1S1
Phone: (902) 628-2257
Fax: (902) 368-2715
E-mail: society@alzpei.ca
Web site: www.alzpei.ca

Federation of Quebec Alzheimer Societies
5165, rue Sherbrook Ouest, Bur. 211
Montreal, QC   H4A 1T6
Phone: (514) 369-7891   Toll free: 1-888-636-6473
Fax: (514) 369-7900
E-mail: info_fqsa@alzheimerquebec.ca
Web site: www.alzheimerquebec.ca

Alzheimer Society of Saskatchewan
2550 – 12th Avenue, Suite 301
Regina, SK   S4P 3X1
Phone: (306) 949-4141   Toll free: 1-800-263-3367
Fax: (306) 949-3069
E-mail: info@alzheimer.sk.ca
Web site: www.alzheimer.sk.ca

Alzheimer's Association National Office (United States)
225 N. Michigan Ave., Fl. 17
Chicago, IL 60601
Phone: (312) 335-8700   Toll free: 1-8001272-3900
Fax: (312) 335-1110
E-mail: info@alz.org
Web site: www.alz.org

Some Helpful Web Sites

Those who are connected to the Internet can keep up with the latest developments on AD as well as communicate with others involved with the disease by accessing various web sites. The list of useful and reliable sites below comes, along with other information, from *Perspectives: A Newsletter for Individuals with AD or a Related Disorder,* published by the University of California at San Diego Alzheimer's Disease Research Center, La Jolla, California.

http://www.alzheimer.ca
The Canadian Alzheimer Society web site has a very helpful and extensive section devoted to persons with dementia, as well as educational material and personal testimonies.

http://www.alzheimers.org.au
This Australian web site has a section devoted to personal cases and an excellent assortment of detailed help sheets on different related topics, which can be downloaded.

http://www.alzheimers.org.uk
This UK site has an excellent site entitled "I Have Dementia," which covers many topics and includes personal experiences and poetry.

http://www.alzheimers.org.uk/westkent

The first local web page designed by people with dementia provides information on the services of this branch and is a voice for such persons.

http://www.alz.org

This web site of the US National Alzheimer Association has a concise but useful section for the person with Alzheimer Disease and a message board for correspondence.

http://www.dasninternational.org

This educational web site and online chat room is designed and organized by the Dementia Advocacy and Support Network (DASN), an international group of individuals with dementia.

http://www.alzheimercafe.co.uk **or**
http://212.250.205.69/contact.htm

This wonderful, innovative program was created by Dr. Bère Miesen in the Netherlands and expanded into the UK in 2000. It helps family members of all ages meet one another in an informal and educational "café" environment. Typically, the two-hour evening is held once a month in a consistent central location. The web site gives information on starting such an Alzheimer Café.